Freedom
from Stuttering

Freedom
from Stuttering

Using Nutrition, Supplements, Natural Strategies, and
Quality Speech Therapy to Rewire the Brain

7 Steps to Being a Fluent Speaker for Life!

PATRICIA A VITEK MCCLAIN

ISBN: 0996128808
ISBN 13: 9780996128803

DEDICATION

This book is dedicated to my husband, Robin,
who always encourages me to spread my wings and fly!

TABLE OF CONTENTS

ACKNOWLEDGEMENTS

A special thank you is extended to my daughter Kaitlyn.
Thank you for always being there for me. You have spent numerous hours listening to me and supporting me through this writing process and in our shared fields.
We share a passion in the field of speech, as speech and language pathology shines brightly in this world.
Kaitlyn, you have a natural gift for helping others in so many ways. You have been inspirational in this process, supported me as my accountability partner, assisted me as editor of this book, and helped make this book a reality. As a published author yourself, I know you understand this heart wrenching process.
Your help is greatly appreciated!

With warm thanks to Krista, Kaitlyn, Heather, Michael, and Halle
Thank you for the patience and support you have exhibited in helping me make my dream come true. I know there have been challenges and yet you have remained on my side and loved me through it all. I hope my book will reach you in a way you never imagined, helping you to know me just a little better, and yourself a little just a little more. Your support means so much to me.
I love you all!
Mom

To my Mom and Dad
For always giving me unconditional love, bringing music and laughter in my life,
and allowing me to be the black sheep of the family,
as I always walked to a different beat.
I miss you and you will always be in my heart.

To my family and friends who helped edit my book:
I will be forever indebted to you for all your time, energy, and help. You have
truly helped me make this dream come true!

My Story

My name is Patricia A. Vitek McClain, M.S., CCC-SLP/L, a Speech and Language Pathologist and Integrative Nutrition Health Coach. I am medically licensed and certified by the American Speech and Hearing Association (ASHA) in speech and language pathology, and a member of the International Association of Health Coaches (IAHC). As a speech and language pathologist, I have worked in both hospitals and schools in both Illinois and California, as well as owning a private practice called Achieving Smiles, where I worked with speech, language, feeding, and literacy skills. I am new to the field of Health Coaching, although health has been a driving force in my life for many years, and I have taken it on in a passionate way. It is my hope to blend my two passions in speech and health in some way, and through this book, my journey begins.

I have been touched by so many amazing individuals, both children and adults, in my profession as a speech and language pathologist, and particularly by the challenges they face on a daily basis. In many therapeutic interventions, we can give a clear bill of health following treatment. Yet there is one particular disorder, that has no cure to date-"stuttering." What makes it more pronounced is the way that it is viewed by society. With new discoveries in the medical aspects of stuttering, there appears to be hope on the horizon, but the cost of current treatments may be far too great, leaving the person who stutters in a no-win situation. This new information touches on the cause for the very first time, even though in both therapy and medicine, the treatment still focuses on the symptoms.

When we know the cause, we can find the cure.

As a Health Coach, I have the amazing opportunity to help others heal them-selves. Whether there is a "cure" or not at this point, together lets seek to heal. Let's embark on a path of discovery of the celebrations in life, the amazing relationships we share, the passions we seek, the physical and mental strength we develop, and grace and solitude that we find in the world and in ourselves. Let's add color to our foods and our life, get a clear picture of our health, and try new and alternative approaches, so that you can be the best YOU that you have the potential to be.

My goal is to guide you through a journey of healing, with a focus on nu-trition and personal health, neuroscience, treatments, and philosophies. Take your health into your own hands.

Don't be afraid to have hope, and make hope a reality.

I am so excited to take this journey with you...

Patricia

A Meaningful Poem About Stuttering,
by Eric Hawkins

When I was born
I was born to fight
The words were trouble
and wouldn't come out right
So I would just walk, in the quiet

I thought long and hard
on the words I said
I would change them around in my head
but the words, were still a mighty fight

Others would laugh
and call me names
They thought my words
were mighty strange
I would just hurt, in the quiet

I dreamed of times
of better days
I dreamed my trouble
would go away
The words were a battle, everyday

The fight of words gave me a life
It gave me a gift
It gave me an eye
That could only be learned, in the quiet.

This poem was written by Eric Hawkins, thanking the Stuttering Association for all they do for those who stutter.
http://www.stutteringhelp.org/content/meaningful-poem-about-stuttering

One

"STUTTERING"

A. Stuttering…What is it?

Stuttering is simply stated by The American Speech and Hearing Association (ASHA) as "affecting the fluency of speech." It sounds simple, however, it is one of the most complex disorders that has emotionally impacted my speech and language clients, as well as most speech and language pathologists. We are continually seeking more information to evaluate and treat this disorder. In addition, understanding what differentiates typical or developmental dysfluency from stuttering challenges speech pathologists and families alike. Parents refer to their child as, "my child is a stutterer," even when the characteristics appear more like a typical developmental dysfluency. There is fear in the intonation as parents mutter their concerns. The word "stuttering" should not be used lightly and/ or as a catch all disorder, and the opposite is also true. "Stuttering" is a complex disorder that involves extensive evaluation and has an extreme emotional impact on the child that stutters, the family, and even the therapists who work with that child.

One of our roles, as speech and language pathologists, is to rule out the difference between typical or developmental dysfluencies and true "stuttering," and in the meantime, even when concern exists, that label should not accompany anyone's initial description of the individual. Labeling a child a "stutterer" may impact how parents and families treat that child, the expectations they place on them, and it may have long-term effects on the parent-child bond. Before the word "stutter" is used to describe any symptoms, extensive evaluation resulting in the diagnostic determination of this label must be first completed.

On the other hand, do not minimize the need for seeking out support from speech and language pathologists early on. There is research to support that most childhood "stuttering" will resolve with early intervention, and only approximately 20% will continue to stutter into adulthood. My contention is that, in the resolved cases, it may possibly never have been true "stuttering" to begin with. Something else may have been interfering with the production of speech or it may have been developmental in nature. Often there are contributing or co-existing factors of speech and language disorders in which dysfluency is a symptom rather than the disorder itself. In any event, a speech and language pathologist trained in both pediatrics and fluency of speech should make that determination.

B. What are the Characteristics of Stuttering?

Stuttering may be evidenced by repetitions of words or parts of words, prolongations of individual sounds in a word, and fillers such as "um" when initiating words or phrases, whether intentional or unintentional. Unusual facial expressions, or blocks, may be evident on the face of the person who stutters. They visually appear to be starting to speak and the words just don't come out. In my experience, speaking appears effortful and the individual who stutters appears breathless. Speech is often very softly spoken and the physical personality of the individual may appear "shy" in conversation.

In my experience, I have noted that easy conversations, even with family or familiar company, may appear effortful and struggled. In this situation, the person who stutters may appear uncomfortable, as does everyone else who is engaged in the conversation. Interestingly, with the same people when watching a football game, the loud and excited cheering will be perfectly fluent in the child that stutters. I have taken this amazing fact into consideration as I develop a treatment plan for the children I treat, which will be discussed further.

C. What Causes Stuttering?

There is not any specific criteria to date that confirms why one person will stutter and another will not. There are certain circumstances that we are aware of that contribute to or influence the development of stuttering. First, we know that a child does not seem to be born a "stutterer." That may raise a question of other influences, such as stress, environmental, and pharmaceutical considerations. We do know that "genetics" come into play since oftentimes, even as much as 60% of the time, there will be another family member in the family line who was known to be a "stutterer." Family influences can contribute to dysfluent speech, particularly as our lives continue to be so high paced with increased expectations, stressful lifestyles, and increased educational and social demands. We often see that dysfluent speech co-exists with other speech and language disorders. What came first, the chicken or the egg? Is it the speech and language disorder that influences the dysfluent speech production, or is it the dysfluent speech that limits speech and language development? More recently, we have discovered that neurophysiology impacts how an individual who stutters processes language. With this in mind, medical management and medications, have been used to remediate stuttering. These findings have opened new hope in the study of fluency at a time when incidence rates are increasing.

Not only are incidence rates in fluency disorders increasing, but there also appears to be a higher prevalence of stuttering in children, implying that other factors may be influencing this disorder. In addition, it has been noted that the incidence in males is twice what it is in females. Then again, our speech and language caseloads have always been predominantly male, so while this finding is noteworthy, it does not seem to be a factor of great merit in determining a cause for stuttering. It may presuppose, however, this co-existing philosophy of speech and language disorders and stuttering. This also explains the reason boys may have a greater incidence.

As a speech and language pathologist, as well as an Integrative Nutrition Health Coach with a Holistic viewpoint, I contend that other factors have a play not only in the development of stuttering, but in the increase in a host of childhood disorders and illnesses. In this era of the industrialized revolution, we must further consider the impact from the air that we breathe, the food that we eat, the water we drink, and the medicinals that we ingest or have injected into us. I believe these factors have a much more dramatic effect on the body, the brain, and may be a large contributing factor to dysfluent speech as you will see when you read further.

> *In conclusion, there is no one direct cause that is attributed to this disorder, but only a set of circumstances that contribute to or influence the development of stuttering.*

D. How is stuttering perceived by families and society as a whole?

Can the quality of life be impacted by the perceptions of others, particularly based on expectations and ideals of the culture? I cannot imagine a world where this cannot be true, as we are a society that depends on human connections. Individuals with autism are subjected to similar perceptions that make them socially detached from others. While the child with autism has difficulty understanding societal social cues to form meaningful relationships, the child who stutters understands the social cues well, which unfortunately are typically negative when they speak, causing many individuals who stutter to withdraw from interactions. This is further complicated as social demands increase in adolescence and as the desire for the opposite sex increases and intimate relationships begin to form.

In my career, I have had referrals from friends of a family who has a child who stutters, and when given the description from the referring family it is presented with a sense of sorrow and sympathy. They say things like, "It's just so sad to see him speak." It would be difficult for them to ever understand the content of what this child is saying because the manner in which it is spoken evokes such sympathy and even discomfort. When the referral is made, I learn nothing more than the fact that this child stutters. The referring family has not been able to reveal any information of who this child is personally. In addition, there is often a sense of contempt, as one may call it, when observing the interaction of a person who stutters out in the community.

When I first began in the field of speech pathology, I took an undergraduate prerequisite course in stuttering. The class was very limited, but there was one assignment that touched my heart forever and has brought me here, to a place of seeking new strategies, and even to the point of writing this book. The assignment was to be a stutterer, on the phone, in a store, and/ or in a restaurant. I made the call first, to place an order by phone and heard a kind voice on the other end. The reaction on the phone as I began to stutter became one of challenge and I couldn't meet the expectations of the person on the other end of the call. There was arrogance and ridicule that was displayed almost immediately as I prolonged and repeated sounds and words. I was cut off before I could actually place the order. Click! They hung up the phone on me. Was the level of ridicule so great because I was believed to be less intelligent than the person I was talking to? Was it so great because I wasn't tolerated? Was I a lower member of a societal class? From the sweet voice on the other end of the phone, to a voice filled with judgment, was what I experienced. When I took my stuttering into a local store, which often employed special needs adults, surprisingly I found similar perceptions. I was in the return line, yet what the interaction evoked felt much greater than any sense of embarrassment and fear that I had ever experienced. It may surprise you that the voice of contempt was far less threatening than the face of contempt, or shall I say faces, as the other people in the store were all focused on me. I was now surrounded by a staring, contempt filled crowd. I never completed the assignment to order in a restaurant, as the impact of this activity had already taken its toll on me. The assignment was complete that day, however the lessons I learned were life-long.

There is also the sympathetic view from families, particularly mothers. I have worked with many families of small children who were dysfluent. There have been a host of situations that impacted these small children, and mostly what I observed was a sense of agony on the part of the mothers. For one reason or the other, they blamed themselves for the disorder, as mothers often take on the problems of the world, bless their hearts. At times, I witnessed a lack of tolerance on the part of parents and families. Yet what concerned me the most, was the impact it had on the bond between family members. When the child became more aware of the families' perceptions, withdrawal compromised their interactions. Overall, this may have long-term effects on relationships and the overall quality of life of the individual who stutters. In addition, it can become a cycle of defeat. When relationships and career or student life are compromised, it is a detriment to overall health and healing, as we will discuss further in this book. One of the primary foods that keep us healthy involves our relationships. Without it, overall health may be compromised.

E. How does stuttering impact the individual who stutters?

We are all faced with challenges, but in all the books I've read and all the people I have spoken with in my career, there is no challenge so great as when speaking fluently isn't an automatic process. We sometimes take for granted the natural ability to walk and talk and the magnitude of development that occurs in the first few years of life. Imagine when there is a disruption in one of those processes. Further imagine, when this disruption of speech fluency evokes such negative perceptions from family, friends, and society as a whole.

The small children I have worked with have varied significantly, from the one who has no idea they stutter to the one that withdraws, as early as 2-3 years old in my practice. Remember that children have speech that is 80% adult-like by 4 years old. When this is disrupted, children and adults alike notice it. Many children who have come to me in these early years of dysfluency, have symptoms that resolve and relationships that are mended with the benefit of speech therapy, not just for the student, but the family as a whole. Then there is that child who has speech therapy for years and years and years. They have reached adolescence and they have "given up." They lose interest in speech therapy and withhold who they really are because they can't speak fluently, yet are faced with families whose fear makes them want more and more therapy so they will be "cured." When I develop a bond with an adolescent child that has been referred to me, I hear of the challenge and utter heartache they experience in all walks of life, individually and even as a member of a family. The mothers continue to hope for a "cure," even when the child, especially at the time of adolescence, has lost all hope.

Parents report that when their child uses the strategies they learn in speech therapy they sound better, yet every moment is a constant reminder of the challenge their child will face in life. They fear the world will never get a chance to know their amazing child. I fear that parents will never get to know their amazing child. Yes, and the child who stutters has often "given up," lost all hope. At the age of adolescence, they don't know that things get better. They are living in a moment that appears to be a life-long sentence. When I first meet the child and their families, the last thing in the world they want is more of the same speech therapy, as the child may take personal blame for not getting better. I often meet with parents first. I tell them that what I will recommend will be unlike anything they have ever done before, and they have to be ready for some unusual recommendations that will impact everyone in the family. Mostly, the one who has to buy into this however, is the child who stutters.

Two

"TRADITIONAL APPROACHES TO TREATMENT"

A. What are the traditional approaches for the treatment of stuttering?

There are a wide variety of approaches that are typically used to treat stuttering. It is not the purpose of this book to discuss and comment on all the various approaches in the context of this chapter, since my purpose is to focus more on a new and more natural approach. In order to explain the reasons for change to a new methodology, there needs to be some comment or clarification on some of the terminology used in the current therapeutic approaches. This will allow the reader to better understand why this new focus of treatment may be considered a more natural approach that treats the cause, rather than the symptoms, and allows for greater empowerment and confidence in the individual. The most difficult factor considered in traditional approaches to treat stuttering (dysfluency) is due to the fact that the symptoms become so significant, the focus of treatment is meant to make the stuttering less severe, use fluent stuttering, and/ or treat the behaviors as if they were fully under the control of the individual, for example. The words often spoken in treatment are things like behavior modification therapy and fluency shaping. There are often terms like easy onset, easy stuttering, fluent stuttering, breath stream management, reduced speech rate, oral motor planning, articulatory contacts, pausing and phrasing, unlearning maladaptive behavior, and self monitoring in the goals of the individual who stutters. Discussions of social and emotional implications are often the first area of treatment, along with treatments for processing auditory language and motor planning. Often, therapy is considered successful when a person speaks fluently with occasional moments of mild stuttering. That sounds successful when it doesn't control the whole person, yet what does it take for the individual to maintain this fluent speech?

In my experience, when I have spoken to adolescents who have spent what feels like a lifetime in speech therapy, and asked how they maintain fluency on a daily basis, I often get a silence, no response. Their confidence in ever being fluent is often diminished. They report that when they use strategies they can be more fluent. Yet, overwhelmingly, they are not consistently using the strategies they were taught. They just talk less. Are they not motivated to be fluent? Don't they care? Must this be a maladaptive behavior that must be reshaped or changed? That seems to be the focus of some of the traditional adolescent treatment plans. I observed many therapists over the years who treat stuttering in adolescents and adults and this seems to be the mindset. As if someone wouldn't want to be fluent, to be able to express themselves in a way that others understand their deepest thoughts. They compromise who they are because of the fear of stuttering. Yet, behavioral, attitudinal, cognitive, and motor therapies continue to be the supported courses of treatment, without considering that these may only be treating the symptoms and not the cause of the stutter.

B. What do other speech and language pathologists think about traditional approaches and new discoveries?

Interviews With Speech Pathologists:
I proposed the following questions to a large population of speech and language pathologists, many of whom I have attended numerous stuttering conferences with. I was surprised by the number of people who respectfully declined my request to respond, feeling that they were not experienced enough to make comment. While I believe that treating even one individual with this disorder qualifies one for comment, I deeply respect their choice to withdraw. To the brave speech pathologists who took on this challenge in the face of sometimes limited success, I thank them for sharing their expertise, successful treatments, comments on the medical model, and their personal joys and sorrows with the clients they have helped over the years. This is a difficult topic, and one that has diverse methodologies of treatments, philosophies, and experiences. It is my hope that after the publishing of this book, there will be an increased number of experienced contributors, parents of children who stutter, and the individuals who stutter, who will come forth to help support others in similar circumstances. This is the first step towards treating the whole individual with a village of support.

I asked my professional associates and friends the following questions:

How do you rate your experience with dysfluency/ stuttering disorders?
What treatment approaches have you used?
How beneficial have these treatments been for your students/ clients?
What obstacles have you faced in working with this population?
Do you believe stuttering can be cured with current interventions?
How do you feel about the medical model and the use of pharmaceuticals in the treatment of stuttering?
Share one experience working with a child or adult with stuttering that has touched your heart.

The experience level ranged from treating 1-2 clients to many clients over many (up to 17) years. Most of the treatment approaches were motor, language, and behaviorally based. One speech pathologist stood out of the norm and shared her experience using voice techniques, particularly for students with blocks. Another speech pathologist with years of experience believed she could successfully remediate stuttering in preschoolers if therapy was implemented right at the onset, and they received a generous amount of time in therapy for the first 2 years. She believed that the ones who persisted faced a combination of issues, including fragile oral motor coordination that could be disrupted by stress, illness, and fatigue. Many speech pathologists recognized the unique nature of the disorder in each of the clients they treated, and they used of variety of individualized treatment methods. They included play-based methods, breathing techniques for reading aloud, and forward flowing speech, as well as voice techniques for clients with blocks or physical concomitants. Some of the obstacles reported were transitions from one school to another, and maintaining support systems along the way. Many reported that self-esteem for older students and self-awareness for younger students were obstacles.

The idea of "curing" a true stutter was not believed to be possible by almost everyone, with the exception of the speech pathologist that was able to remediate stuttering prior to kindergarten and with her own child. The idea of this early remediation may suggest the possibility that there were other co-existing or influencing factors to the dysfluency. There is also the consideration of developmental dysfluency, which remediates on its own no later than by 10 years old. Interestingly some SLP's had not heard of the medical model and several others who were aware of the medical model shared positive results from pharmaceutical treatments. One speech pathologist reported a student who made dramatic improvements in overall fluency with medication years ago, however later suffered from psychosis. Another speech pathologist has a friend on medication showing remarkable results. Few commented on the other symptoms that erupted from pharmaceuticals, but were exceedingly impressed with the improvements in fluent speech. Psychosis, depression, low libido, and withdrawal have all been mentioned as side effects to this treatment. Dr. Gerald Maguire discusses the proposed and possible benefits of drugs to treat stuttering with the down side of negative and significant side-effects, dosing complications, and limited long-term use possibilities. (http://www.stuttering-help.org/genetic-and-neurological-factors-stuttering)

Finally, I was touched by the personal stories that were shared- thank you all. They included endearing success stories of their own children and clients who have touched their hearts along the way. Therefore, I end these interviews with a quote from a speech and language pathologist that held such joy and positive approaches with her students and her responses radiated with hope. This particular clinician bonded well with a particular student who each week, shared all the strategies he tried in a variety of situations. She spoke for all of us with the words she used to conclude her interview.

"These are the moments that I sit in awe, grateful for the journeys that I get to call "work" on a daily basis."

We are truly blessed to work in a profession that can make a difference in individuals, families, and the world.

To the individuals who stutter:
It is my hope that if even one individual finds acceptance and joy in himself, and maybe even possibly can be "cured," my time writing this book will be well spent.

To the families of the individual who stutters:
I hope this book builds understanding, compassion, and healing for you all. Look past the stuttering and discover the whole child within.

And to my associates, the amazing speech pathologists around the world:
All your individualized efforts are recognized, no matter what philosophy or treatment protocol you support.

And to the world:
May you someday soon accept the differences in each of us with no judgment.

With sincere thanks to you all…

C. What are the new medically-based discoveries?

Recent breakthroughs in the field of medicine have made claims that there may be some aspect for a medical basis of stuttering. The focus is on the use of medication to treat stuttering, yet there has been no claim that this in any way will be a cure, or that this in any way should replace traditional therapies.

The medical aspects of stuttering intrigued me immensely a few years ago following a fluency conference on the topic of medical management of stuttering, presented by Dr. Gerald A. Maguire (gerald.maguire@uci.edu), where he focused on the pharmacologic treatments used to treat stuttering. Following that conference, I was rejuvenated with new hope in finding a possible cause of stuttering, and I have been researching and trying new approaches based on these new findings. The medical discovery considered a hypothesis of excessive dopamine, since it was found that most subjects studied shared one common characteristic: an overproduction of dopamine. It was also suggested that it may not just be the overproduction of dopamine, but there may be a break in the dopamine pathway, in addition to an over-production of dopamine. The course of treatment, or medical management, was really the focus of this conference, more than the fact that this may be a causal factor for dysfluency. The use of psychotropic drugs, typically used to treat a variety of mental health issues, were given to teens in lower amounts with the focus of treating stuttering. Disorders of schizophrenia for example, involve the dopamine pathways, so it was logical to consider these medications in treating a related dopamine-based disorder of a much less severe nature with similar medications in reduced dosages. In very simple terms, the research showed that with medication, the stuttering improved, but the personalities of the teens given this medication were considerably more iso-lated and withdrawn. They were noted to have a loss of sex drive and an inability to focus. Although, I am tremendously encouraged by the medical aspects of stuttering in determining causal factors of this disorder, it seems to me that with or without the medication, the individuals who stutter were still forced to compromise who they are.

At the time, my clients with dysfluency were of preschool and elementary age. I posed a question to the presenters about what we may be able to do more naturally, with food or supplements, for younger children. There were no studies or even consideration at this age, and this topic, not being pharmaceutical in nature, was quickly dismissed. This did not stop my interest in this area. As I researched in greater detail, I found foods that increase and decrease neurotransmitters, such as dopamine. I began exploring foods that would decrease dopamine, for example, if this was one of the culprits influencing dysfluent speech patterns. Protein-rich foods tend to increase dopamine and norepinephrine, the fight or flight neurotransmitters that increase alertness and concentration, and also involve the fight or flight reaction times. Since sleep and mood were often impacted, I considered complex carbohydrates to increase serotonin, the calming neurotransmitter. For example, buckwheat, which is rich in tryptophan, is also a precursor to serotonin which regulates sleep and mood. (http://www.lef.org/Magazine/2008/4/Why-Aging-People-Become-Depressed-Fatigued-And-Overweight/Page-01)

I recommended eating buckwheat in the evening to observe the benefits of the calming effect it may have on the children who stutter. Improved sleep and mood are necessary factors to improve the focus and concentration necessary to improve on anything we do, as well as in improving overall health.

D. Where do we go from here?

As I begin this introduction of the gut-brain connection in conjunction with these new medical discoveries, I want to take a moment to comment on the new horizon ahead of us in treating stuttering. This is an important time in finding the cause of stuttering, and the dopamine hypothesis is a wonderful beginning. Look now to the differences in traditional medicine and in the functional medicine model. In traditional medicine, the medical community looks to pharmaceuticals to address these new findings, and in particular the symptoms of stuttering. We recognize the side effects of pharmaceuticals may be more problematic than the stuttering itself for some. On the other hand, the functional medicine doctor looks for the cause of health issues and approaches treatment with food as medicine. The functional and naturopathic medicine community recognizes the gut-brain connection, and in particular the relationship between digestive health and cognitive/ mental health issues. Dr. Chris Kresser reports that "the gut-brain axis is one of the most important and least recognized factors in human health." (http://chriskresser.com/the-healthy-skeptic-podcast-episode-9)

As we begin this journey, consider the relationship between the gut and the brain.

Three

IN DEFENSE OF FOOD,
IN DEFENSE OF OUR YOUTH

Living in a World with Processed and
Genetically Modified Foods

A. What do we mean by processed foods?

First let me say that a picture is worth a thousand words. Close your eyes and visualize a large supermarket. Around the periphery, we typically find fruits, vegetables, dairy, and meats, otherwise known as "real foods." Real foods can sometimes be processed. For example, we may take a steak and grind it into hamburgers and we may churn butter from the cream that separates from the milk. In any event, in this type of processing, nothing is added to the product so that it may still be considered to be "real food."

Now picture that large supermarket again. After sculpting the periphery for real food, note that the entire middle of the store is made up of the big bad wolf of products-chemically processed foods. These foods are chemically processed from refined and/ or artificial ingredients. When I further speak of "processed foods," this reference is to the chemically processed foods in our world, as will be further discussed.

The only benefit to chemically processed foods is to the financial bottom line of big business. They are cheap products, made to taste in a way that is pleasing and addictive, and they consistently use inexpensive ingredients, often genetically modified ingredients, making these products cash cows for big businesses. They are also marketed in ways that appeal to our sense of convenience. Rather than coming home, scanning through the lonely items on the refrigerator shelves, and thinking about how you can make something taste half good, just opening a bag or package is often a preferred choice for most. It's simple and convenient. It's ready to go, takes minutes to prepare, and always tastes the same.

A snack that I would occasionally indulge in many years ago was a popular cheesy, salty, crunchy snack. It was a guilty pleasure for sure. Yet as my label reading improved, I began to wonder what real ingredients were in any of these guilty pleasures that may make their way past my lips.

I recently picked up a package of this popular snack item on the grocery store shelves and checked out the ingredients and any packaging changes since my days of indulgence (see below). The picture below was what I found on the internet: "MADE WITH ALL NATURAL OIL— WE GROW THE BEST SNACKS ON EARTH." In evaluating the ingredient list, I made every attempt to simply find anything that was actually "grown." Most of the ingredients were unfamiliar and some were even difficult to pronounce.

My cheesy, salty, and crunchy snack days are over for sure. After eating real foods for so many years, they become the true guilty pleasures (without the guilt of course), making the chemically processed foods far less appealing and in fact, are often now an awful tasting proposition for me. There is an after taste that sends a negative message to my brain. Keep away!

Ingredients: Enriched Corn Meal (Corn Meal, Ferrous Sulfate, Niacin, Thiamin Mononitrate, Riboflavin, and Folic Acid), Vegetable Oil (Corn, Canola, Soybean, and/or Sunflower Oil), Flamin' Hot Seasoning (Less than 2% of the Following: Maltodextrin [Made From Corn], Salt, Sugar, Monosodium Glutamate, Yeast Extract, Citric Acid, Artificial Color [Red 40 Lake, Yellow 6 Lake, Yellow 6, Yellow 5], Partially Hydrogenated Soybean and Cottonseed Oil, Sunflower Oil, Cheddar Cheese [Milk, Cheese Cultures, Salt, Enzymes], Onion Powder, Whey, Whey Protein Concentrate, Garlic Powder, Corn Syrup Solids, Natural Flavor, Buttermilk, Sodium Diacetate, Sodium Caseinate, Lactic Acid, Disodium Inosinate, Disodium Guanylate, Skim Milk), and Salt.

CONTAINS MILK INGREDIENTS.

MADE WITH
ALL NATURAL OIL

WE GROW THE BEST
SNACKS ON EARTH®

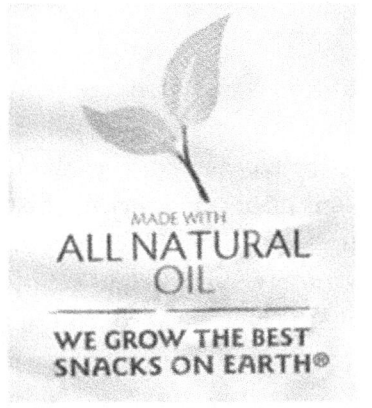

B. What about the fats?

Our bodies are lean mean fighting machines, but when the machine is oiled with poor quality oil, the chance of the engine running efficiently or for an extended time is unlikely. That is the first of the reasons why chemically processed foods are bad for us. It's the oil. Most oils in processed foods are refined vegetable oils which contain excessive omega 6 fats, and are often laced with cheap, refined, and hydrogenated vegetable oils: Hello-Trans Fats!

For example, lets also add Canola oil into the mix. It seems like every product now contains canola oil, and on every cooking show it's used in every recipe they make. What's a canola? And what exactly is an organic canola? Canola is processed from the rapeseed plant, which is 100% toxic to humans. In a laboratory, they converted it into only a slightly toxic oil, but by whose definition? Since it originated in a lab, there were no farmers, pesticides, or fertilizers. Does the omission of this mean something is organic? The byproduct of this process is somewhere in the neighborhood of gasoline fumes, and it contains a high sulfur content, making it turn rancid quickly. In Canola oil, the omega 3's are converted into trans fats, which depletes the vitamin E necessary for optimal heart function. Stick with coconut oil, extra virgin olive oil, and even avocado oil, the heart healthy alternatives.

C. What about the sugars-particularly High Fructose Corn Syrup?

Most processed foods are very high in sugars, particularly high fructose corn syrup, made from genetically modified corn. Most of the processed foods on the shelves contain large amounts of sugars and high fructose corn syrup. I found it shocking that the first ingredient in many infant formulas was high fructose corn syrup-Yes! Shocking! No wonder breast fed babies never fall into the norms on the weight graphs at the pediatrician's office. Breast milk doesn't have the high sugar content of formula, so the growth rate will be more natural and stable. Sugar has been tied to all of the leading diseases in our country. On average, an American consumes 150 pounds of sugar a year. Sugar makes you crave more sugar-it's addictive. Want to see the weight come off? Don't worry about quality fats. Just worry about your sugar intake.

D. What about artificial ingredients?

Look again at the ingredient list above for my cheesy and salty indulgence of the past. Look at any snack label you find on the shelf of the grocery store. I would wager to believe that you won't know what half the ingredients are, and you may be unable to pronounce some of them. Is this really what you want to put in your body? Is this really what you want to feed your children? I dare you to find a processed food that has less than 5 ingredients. I try to shoot for an occasional 3 ingredient guilty pleasure, but they are few and far between.

E. What about refined carbohydrates?

Refined carbohydrates, as in grains (cereals, breads, etc.) cause blood sugar spikes and increased insulin levels, which are followed by a crash. The crash causes you to crave more sugar, and so the cycle begins again. It's exhausting, not to mention, the negative health effects of this yoyo impact on the body. White is not the new black, so avoid the white flours in particular. Each American today eats almost 146 pounds of flour a year, including wheat flour. The interesting note is that flour spikes insulin more than sugar. I often hear people say, "I am not a sugar addict, I just like the breads, bagels, and pasta." In general, grains or heavily processed foods contain higher carbohydrate contents. In the body, these carbohydrates convert to glucose. When there is excess glucose, it gets stored as fat. Excess glucose, insulin spikes, and insulin resistance, are detrimental to the brain. In particular, the cells begin to prevent the uptake of amino acids, necessary food for the neurotransmitters in the brain.

In summary, chemically processed foods lead to negative health consequences and provide a benefit only to big business. This leads me now to genetically modified foods. The game changes for the worse.

F. What is genetic modification (GMO's)?

Genetic modification is done in a laboratory, and it involves the transfer of genetic material to plants or animals. This is done in such a way so to create a species that has mutated into something that can withstand large amounts of herbicides, and even create pesticide toxins within the cells of the plant itself. The seed becomes a pesticide producer. There is concern of allergies, disease, and compromised immunological function, of which the long term effects are unknown. The Institute for Responsible Technology, www.resonsibletechnology.org/healthrisks, describes some of the hazards of consuming GMO's and provides resources to start buying non-GMO products and prevents genetically engineering our food sources.

The most genetically modified foods, up to 90% in our food supply, are soy, corn, canola, alfalfa, zucchini and yellow squash, sugar beets, and milk. Soy is the most genetically modified food in this country and 85% of the corn grown in the US is genetically modified. (Carolyne Young, Huffington Post-12/03/2013)

G. *What's the big deal anyway?*

Take for example, corn. The majority of corn grown in the United States today is genetically modified. It produces a Bt toxin, which causes an insect's gut to explode when taking a bite. Now we are much larger than an insect, but we also eat a whole ear of corn, or more! There are about 800 kernels on an average ear of corn. Imagine that if one kernel destroys the gut of an insect, what do you think 800 kernels will do to a human being? I am often hearing about "leaky gut" and "IBS-Irritable bowel syndrome." There are no definitive diagnoses, yet it is interesting that there are a host of new symptoms creeping up that are now so common we have whole new categories of gut illnesses. In addition, when the gut is penetrated into the lymph system, it has the possibility of reaching other organs and some of the most important organs in the body-the brain, the adrenals, and the heart. We also face an incredibly increased incidence of fertility problems, which correlated to the decreased fertility of animals who were fed GMO foods.

I remember in the 1990's, there was news that the US created a seed that could withstand droughts in countries like Africa. My kids and I were overjoyed at the prospects of feeding starving countries. It sounded too good to be true, and like anything else that is too good to be true, it was. If I had any idea that we were feeding a starving population something that was a nutrient depleted and pesticide producing food, I would have done everything in my power to stop it.

Advertising made this seed invention sound like it was too good to be true, when in reality, we were growing toxic substances disguised as food. Advertising was persuasively manipulating logical thought, and this continues today. There have been isolated products, such as cigarettes, where advertising was restricted for children, however the potential to target Monsanto, *the main producer of genetically modified crops and seeds in the world* and one of the wealthiest companies in the world, has been met with great opposition. The chemical giants in our country have now taken to using a back door to advertise to our youth, in our textbooks. Under the science of biotechnology, they are doing nothing more than attempting to brainwash them to secure the future of a chemically processed world. It's advertising at its most deceptive!

H. What is the impact of Grain and Sugar on the brain?

Our health is not something that we tend to outwardly seek, until we are faced with a scary diagnosis in a cold, white doctor's office. As a speech and language pathologist, brain injuries dominate our profession, whether a trauma to the brain, stroke, aneurism, attention deficit, etc., or even when no identifiable cause is evident. In the convenient oriented lifestyle we live in, and faced with media that influences our logical thought, there are no worries. There is always a pill to solve all of our problems. Yet what is the real problem? We have a medical community who fails to seek the underlying cause of a problem, as they have been conditioned from medical school on, to prescribe a pill. In most medical programs, nutrition and lifestyle are not even in the curriculum, yet we know today that diet and lifestyle have a significant impact on our overall health. And particularly grain and sugar, have a detrimental effect on our body, and especially our brain. Dr. David Perlmutter, in *Grain Brain,* shares that our brain's ultimate destiny is not in our genes, but rather in the food's we eat. He reveals that grain and sugar on the brain create silent inflammation which can be deadly.

Sugar has been proven to harm both the structure and function of the brain. High glucose has been associated with decreased memory and shrinking of the hippocampal regions of the brain, yet even glucose levels from non-vegetable carbohydrates can be as problematic. Cognition, memory, attention, depression, and a host of other disorders are associated with sugar intake. It would be simple if we just saw the ingredient "sugar" on the labels to keep away from these addictive treats that we crave. But sugar is hidden in terms like high fructose corn syrup, fructose, glucose, sucrose, dextrose, and the list goes on. Remember that "sugar" may be the grain based sugars and starches as well, and even the real fruit sugars can cause similar effects. There are almost 60 names for 'sugar' in the ingredient lists we find today, and we continually are increasing the sugar numbers in our food supply. Just think, if the average man, woman, and child in America today eats 150 pounds of sugar and 146 pounds of flour, which equates to sugar in the impact it has on the body, that is almost 300 pounds of 'sugar' in a year. It doesn't seem like there can be room for anything else.

The worst sugar of all is high fructose corn syrup (HFCS) because of the significant spike it causes in blood sugar, tripling the effect of even table sugar on the glycemic load. HFCS is also most likely made from genetically modified corn. That first sweet taste immediately triggers the sweet reward system in the brain, a system of electrical impulses that instill cravings and tolerance for sugar. You lose all control and sweetness dominates your cravings. It's an addictive element that has been compared to cocaine, winning out as the most addictive drug. There are also receptors in the gut that send signals to the brain to produce more insulin for all this sugar intake. It results in sugar shock and you have excess insulin in the body. This opens the door for a host of health issues not limited to diabetes, but circulation problems, high blood pressure, increased triglycerides, inflammation, and even possibly cancer.

Yet the biggest area of concern in terms of our discussions herein, is the fact that too much sugar can spike dopamine and set it into excess. The common link in the current medical research is that individuals who stutter often have an excess of dopamine as well as breaks in the dopamine pathways. Can sugar be the driving force behind the increased incident rates of this disorder in children? In general, children today consume an overwhelming amount of sugar. It would seem that the relationship between sugar and dopamine should warrant further research in treating stuttering at the very minimum. Hmmm... yet the sugar industry is a big political force in our country. Big Pharma will continue to tout the magic pill. The medical community continues to treat the symptoms-you know, the smoke without the fire. Therefore, I am writing this book, so that together we can take a position in defense of our food, and in defense of our children. It won't be an easy task.

Four

Finding and Treating the Cause of Stuttering with Nutrition and Supplements

Introduction

When we think of our overall food intake, most of the focus in America today is about appearance. Being thin becomes the ideal in the materialistic world we live in today, as evidenced by the thousands of diet books on the best sellers list. The promise of ultimate physiques has driven a culture to seek unachievable thinness without any focus on health. There is an inner beauty that glows on the outside when we focus our efforts on healing this lean mean fighting machine we have, and a glow that radiates from head to toe when we focus on the health of the "whole" individual.

Health and well being means that we must focus on both primary and secondary foods, or rather the *balance* of primary and secondary foods. As an Integrative Nutrition Health Coach, I have healed myself in so many ways with the guidance of my educational program and achieved balance in my life. This involves so much more than just the food we eat. Primary foods include positive and thriving relationships, passionate careers, strength and energy from physical exercise, and peace from the conventions of spirituality. The Institute for Integrative Nutrition teaches, *"When primary food is balanced and satiated, your life feeds you, making what you actually eat secondary."*

http://www.integrativenutrition.com/blog/2008/03/26/primary-food It's the balance of both primary and secondary foods, that leads to optimal health and well being. Knowing that when we are fed with primary foods, secondary foods just don't seem as important. When primary foods are in balance, cravings seem to slide by the wayside, addictions are just a word in the dictionary, and control is a force of energy within us. So as we take on the nutritional aspects of this program, be reminded that your energy force will come from the "whole" you, not just the fuel that we put in our bodies. Although as indicated above, there is a guiding principle to heal the primary foods first, and the secondary foods will just fall into place. In the event of stuttering, relationships may be challenged, the motivation to exercise may be fought with resistance, fulfillment as a student or in a career may suffer, and how can the individual who stutters see the beauty and grace in a world that finds so much discomfort in his or her presence? We have become a nation who has made great strides in being colorblind when it comes to skin tone, yet judgment prevails in so many other ways. Women today are still struggling for equality. Overweight individuals are assumed to have no willpower or control. The list goes on. Individuals who stutter may experience judgment and prejudices in their own way.

Take a moment here to breathe and reflect on the gifts of acceptance and compassion as we take notice of differences in each other.
Celebrate the difference....

In the case of stuttering, as the causal factor to the decline in primary food, I contend that we start with using food as medicine to treat the possible causal factors, while focusing on quality speech therapy and health coaching to achieve balance in both the primary and secondary foods. For now, we will begin our point of focus on secondary foods, since stuttering has a neurological element of health concerns that requires immediate attention.

Let's begin by using Food as Medicine!

How do we Heal the Brain with Nutrition?

The recent medical findings linking excess or disrupted dopamine to be a possible cause of stuttering have been the most encouraging piece of information to date. Dopamine is a neurotransmitter in the brain, which also has a genetic component. Healing the brain and combating the genes becomes the first critical response we must consider. By healing the brain with food as medicine, we can improve all neurotransmitters in the brain, and when we improve in one area, other areas often improve as well. Stuttering is a symptom of a more complex problem in the central nervous system and the brain. By providing the necessary vitamins and minerals to the brain or nourishing the brain, our unique body will have the power to heal itself. It's interesting, but we can do an extensive amount of damage to our bodies, and somehow the body always recovers, until the damage gets too extensive and the lean mean fighting machine has no fight left. So lets give the brain the nutrients and essential fats, while simultaneously decreasing inflammation. Note that our genes do not define us either, and we can defy our genes with nutrition.

To heal the brain, there is a necessary level of nutrients and antioxidants required which we can only get from food. Forget all the processed foods, the genetically modified foods, the sugar, the refined grains, the artificial ingredients, and the bad fats, and lets get down to business...*Real Food!* What is real food? How will we know it when we see it? How can we be more savvy at discerning the differences between real and fake foods? Let's make it easy.

...Real Food

First, are we forced to eliminate foods?

In the last chapter, we presented the current problems with food today that play a role in our nation's declining health, and particularly children's health. Therefore, by targeting the removal of processed foods, bad fats, insulin spiking sugars, artificial ingredients, refined carbohydrates, and GMO's, we will no doubt improve our overall health, but you may be seriously questioning, "what's left to eat?" This sentence was not meant to be shocking by any means, but a way of increasing awareness of exactly what we are putting in our mouths, and the impact this may possibly have on our overall health and the health of our children- whether now or later. I personally know the challenge we face to make significant changes in our lives and in the lives of our families, no matter what that may be. Often, food tends to be comforting and we seek it for reasons other than nourishment, or even consider the possible impact it may have on our health. We are often more concerned about how much weight we may gain, or how many calories this product has! From personal experience, I can tell you that a simple 30 day plan of clean, real food will change your attitude about what you eat forever, and even your waistline will thank you. You will find taste buds that you never knew you had. You will discover colors again that will burst with flavor and various textures in your mouth. You will learn to eat real food, maybe for the first time in your life. And you will learn to recognize your body and what it's saying to you.

In this book, I am not asking you to eliminate foods, but instead to include real foods into your diet. This lean mean fighting machine that you have has an amazing ability to recover. Your body is always seeking good health and a little goes a long way. So instead of making this a plan of *elimination*, let's make it a plan of *inclusion*. I challenge you here and now to add in a beautiful array of color to your life. Forget about, or maybe just minimize the whites and the browns, and seek the reds, blues, purples, greens, oranges, yellows.... Although I am specifically targeting color in our foods, a little color in life would be a marvelous thing!

Why should we forget or minimize most of the whites?

In the last chapter, I spoke about sugar and refined grains on the brain. I consider them equally detrimental to our health, and particularly to the neurotransmitters in the brain that we are working to balance for optimal fluent speech. Almost all products with the exception of the periphery of the store contain one or both of these ingredients. Remember that dopamine plays a big role in stuttering, and sugar, in any form, increases dopamine. When too much sugar is added, it can play havoc with dopamine. Remember that sugar craves more sugar, so when the withdrawal symptoms occur, remember to include some color. The more color you add, the less white you will crave. Think of beautiful berries, pink grapefruits, colorful kales, and an array of peppers. Who needs the whites anyway? That is unless whites are in those fabulous fruits and vegetables.

For a variety of nutrients and benefits, we need to eat the colors of the rainbow.
It's a colorful rainbow of nutrients!

Did you know that the colors of fruits and vegetables actually have nutrients that target specific health benefits in the body? There are several books and a new one releasing soon on using color as a cure. For example, someone dear to me suffered a heart attack a few years ago and needed to repair the damage it caused. He asked me to present at his company during Heart Health Month, which is February. Part of my presentation included foods that were protective against heart attacks. It would make sense that "red," as in cranberries, tomatoes, and apples, may give the heart and blood a colorful boost!

Red fruits and vegetables are high in lycopene, a powerful antioxidant. They are helpful in blood building and supporting energy.

Purple fruits and vegetables are protectors of the nervous system- not only the brain, eyes, and skin, but also the digestive system, and may even support healthy blood pressure. They are high in phytochemicals. Sometimes the colors are more of a blue/ purple, and they are rich in powerful antioxidants. The *blues* are particularly beneficial for one's throat and the thyroid.

Orange fruits and vegetables are high in vitamin C and beta-carotene. It is an anti-inflammatory color. It benefits your immune system, eyes, and even blood sugar regulation. Orange fruits and vegetables are very important to the lungs, esophagus, and stomach.

Green fruits and vegetables are neutralizers. Their dark green pigment is from chlorophyll, which is a known detoxifier of the liver. The lighter *yellow greens* are high in lutein, which is important for eye health.

Even *black* and *white* fruits and vegetables have beneficial properties. Now the point here is that if you are trying to heal your heart, don't eat just red fruits and vegetables. What this idea emphasizes is that variety is the spice of life, as the key to achieving better health is really about "balance." If each of these colors has properties of healing, then what is the synergistic benefit of an array of colors? In other words, 2 + 2 = 10! My mother carried around a color wheel with her when ever she shopped for clothes. She would only buy colors that complimented her look. She taught me that I could look fabulous in certain colors and drab in others. Well, mom, this is one way that I can enjoy an array of colors, and I will look amazing in all of them!

Real Food #1 Fruits and vegetables
Consume a diet rich in color! Nourish your brain!

In order to avoid the chemicals and pesticides, the optimal fruits and vegetables one should consume would probably be grown in your backyard. Unfortunately, this is mostly a thing of the past. I have had my difficulties growing my own fruits and vegetables; however I have found that I am the master of herbs and peppers! So when our green thumb is lacking or gardening is only something our grand-mothers did, we need to consider a continuum from best to worst in this category. Farmers markets can be as good as growing fruits and vegetables in your own backyard, and you are eating the freshest of all farm grown products. Sometimes, they may not have the stamp of an organic farm from the USDA because the cost is just too high. These farmers practice organic farming, and they are able to offer you a lower price by not paying this fee. Know your farmers. Organic fruits and vegetables, and local fruits and vegetables, are the best choices you can buy today. Next in line are conventional fruits and vegetables, and last is genetically modified fruits and vegetables. Organic fruits and vegetables are at a premium and are not always something affordable to everyone. Unfortunately, the organic agricultural industry has not been supplemented financially by our government. It is my hope for this to change in the very near future. In the meantime, consider buying *seasonal* organic fruits and vegetables. They are fresher for sure, may even be local, and they are definitely cheaper. Follow the *Dirty Dozen, Clean 15* rules. Some fruits and vegetables, even with increased pesticides sprayed on them, do not absorb as much into the meat of the product. These are ways to afford organics or to not worry as much when you must buy conventional. Conventional fruits and vegetables have been sprayed with significantly more pesticides than organic fruits and vegetables. The *Dirty Dozen, Clean 15* will give more information to view the healthiest and riskiest of these options and allow the buyer to prioritize their purchases, even on a budget. This information is released by the Environmental Working Group (http://wwwewg.org/foodnews/) in the "Shopper's Guide to Pesticides in Produce." I have included the list below. I wash my fruits and vegetables, even the organic ones by soaking them in a vinegar and water bath for 20 minutes. Vinegar pulls much of the pesticide residue from the products, and interestingly, even my organic berries stay fresher longer. Last, we have the genetically modified fruits and vegetables. While I believe any fruits and vegetables are better than no fruits and vegetables, I am hesitant regarding GMO's, particularly when trying to heal the brain. When healing, we don't want to confuse the body with increased and damaging chemicals, since the seeds of these plants are pesticide producers. The pesticides are actually in the fruit or vegetable, so it cannot be washed off. In addition, GMO foods have been reported to be nutrient deficient when compared to their organic counterparts. We need all the nutrients we can get to heal the brain, without any conflicting chemicals contributing to problems. So grow your own, or buy organic and/ or conventional and give them a good wash!

Dirty dozen and the Clean 15

Dirty Dozen, plus	Clean 15
Apples	Avocados
Strawberries	Sweet corn
Grapes	Pineapples
Celery	Cabbage
Peaches	Sweet peas (frozen)
Spinach	Onions
Sweet bell peppers	Asparagus
Nectarines (imported)	Mangoes
Cucumbers	Papayas
Cherry tomatoes	Kiwi
Snap peas (imported)	Eggplant
Potatoes	Grapefruit
Plus: hot peppers and domestic blueberries	Cantaloupe (domestic)
	Cauliflower
	Sweet potatoes

How do I identify the differences between organic, conventional, and genetically modified fruits and vegetables?

Organic codes on fruits and vegetables-5 digits starting with a 9 Genetically modified fruits and vegetables-5 digits starting with an 8 Conventional fruits and vegetables-4 digits usually starting with a 4 (occasionally other four digit numbers if the fruits or vegetables come from other countries. Then we really also can't be confident in the number, as other countries employ various number systems and have different agricultural policies.)

Real Food #2- Meats, organ meats, fish, saturated fats, bone broth Consume a diet rich in grass fed meats, wild caught fish, and coconuts and avocados for your cognitive strength!

As a vegetarian for many years due to my sadness of the inhumanity of animals, I hesitated to include meat in my diet. After several years, my health started to decline. My cholesterol and triglycerides were elevated, my C-reactive protein was in the dangerous range, I received a diagnosis of Celiac's disease, and I was classified in a pre-diabetic state with blood sugars that were continuing to rise. I was fatigued and faced with autoimmune reactions. My lean mean fighting machine was losing the battle. For some, they will do well on a vegetarian diet, provided they are optimizing their protein intake. For me, while I was healthy for a number of years eating this way, my body was changing and letting me know I needed to take a different path. If I kept up my vegetarian and high carbohydrate lifestyle in spite of what my body was telling me, I expect the future would be dismal.

Listen to what your body is telling you!

What I found most interesting was that as a vegetarian, I craved red meat. There were times I would have done anything for a steak, but this would pass, and then the cravings would increase. Also as a vegetarian, my protein intake was definitely lacking. The amazing brain had this funny way of letting me know I was protein deficient, by triggering a craving for steak. It was letting me know that this lean mean fighting machine needed meat for survival. Listen to what your body is telling you. Brain food includes proteins of grass fed beef, organ meat, and especially avocados and coconuts. Organ meats are also high in CoQ10, which increases the energy in the brain and aids in defending the body against toxicity. Add bone broth, although not a protein or fat magnet, it is very high in the necessary mineral content.

Amino acids happen to be the building blocks of protein. Therefore the foods that have the highest content of amino acids are those that are the highest in protein, such as lean meats, poultry, seafood, eggs, and dairy products. Of the plant-based foods that have a high protein and amino acid content are quinoa and soy. I hesitate with eating soy due to the fact that in excess of 90% of all soy produced today is genetically modified. Beans, nuts, and seeds have high protein contents, but lack some of the essential amino acids necessary for the brain.

Interestingly, many of my adult years were driven by the low fat, low cholesterol era. I was told to eat egg white omelets, and to avoid meats, and especially coconuts because it was the big bad wolf of saturated fats. What I find so alarming is that our brains are made up of mostly fat-particularly saturated fat, and cholesterol, so to limit these sources, meant I was starving my brain of the necessary nutrients it needed to function optimally. My brain today is rich in high quality fats and dietary cholesterol. Yes mom, I now love eggs, especially the yolks, and I use butter from pasture-raised cows to fry the eggs! My mom would appreciate this because she fried our eggs in bacon fat, and she would never leave out the yolk. Also noteworthy are the other factors such as cardio health that benefits from saturated fat and many other bodily functions, including bone health, as well as liver, lungs, and immune functions.

Time to nourish the brain with quality saturated fats!

Real Food #3 Dairy
Consume raw dairy from pasture-raised animals,
a nutritional powerhouse for the brain!

Most dairy products today are pasteurized and even ultra pasteurized. This process is meant to preserve shelf life, however it destroys vital nutrients. I have had difficulty finding raw milk even today, yet in Europe you will even find it in vending machines. Raw milk comes from happy pasture raised cows. It makes sense that cows that graze on grass will have a higher nutrient base.

Pasteurization depletes quality vitamins and minerals and leaves the milk nutrient deficient. When I consumed pasteurized dairy in the past, I experienced bouts of headaches and sinus mucus, and almost everyone I know today is lactose intolerant. When we switched to raw milk, the symptoms that made them lactose intolerant and the headaches and mucus I displayed, were no longer a problem. Don't be afraid of raw dairy. There are natural enzymes and probiotics that may have positive benefits on overall health. Although I personally prefer coconut milk as opposed to milk from animals (cows and goats) in general, I enjoy a little raw cream in my morning coffee and raw cheeses like gruyere and parmesan on occasion.

What about supplements?

At my last visit with my naturopathic doctor, he informed me of the nutrition class he was teaching in medical school. He had given the med students the assignment of creating a one-day food plan that met the recommended daily allowance (RDA) of all vitamins and minerals. What he wanted the students to learn from this exercise was that the RDA was unattainable with diet alone. He explained to them that the guidelines for the recommended daily allowance was accepted during WWII, and was formed as a nutritional guideline for the military. It was based on the diet of West Point Students, who at the time were only elite males. In other words, the standards didn't represent the average population, but a very small-defined group. The point of sharing this story was the fact that it is nearly impossible for an individual to achieve the RDA with food alone, and for most of the population, supplements are necessary for supporting optimal health. In addition, the nutrient density of our fruits and vegetables varies greatly in our choices and the nutrient density of the soil it's grown in.

Now the population today, consumes a diet of nutrient deficient food, such as pasteurized milk, genetically modified fruits and vegetables, and industrialized meats, for example. Diets are generally rich in carbohydrates, particularly sugar and grains.

What is the brain to do?

Rather than shooting blindly, I have recommended that my clients test their neurotransmitters in the brain. We know that individuals who stutter have excess or interrupted dopamine cycles. Let's know for sure what is going on. Neurotransmitters impact many functions in the brain and, when they are out of balance, can cause adverse symptoms.

There are inhibitory neurotransmitters, which means that they calm the brain, and excitatory neurotransmitters, which means that they stimulate the brain. Dopamine is the only neurotransmitter that is thought to be both inhibitory and excitatory. It is a very important neurotransmitter that when in excess or disrupted can play havoc on the brain. The medical community has linked the dopamine hypothesis as a possible causal factor for stuttering. Once we know what neurotransmitters are out of balance, we can begin providing more targeted nutritional benefits and supplementing slowly and carefully to balance the brain. Health coaches need to work hand in hand with integrative or naturopathic doctors, knowledgeable in both the neurotransmitter systems of the brain and the impact of excessive or disrupted dopamine, to balance the neurotransmitters carefully. It is preferred the doctors have a knowledge of nutrition as well. In the clients I have worked with who stutter, I have observed not only an excess of dopamine, however, a depletion of other neurotransmitters such as serotonin and norepinephrine. Stress can deplete neurotransmitters, as well as stimulants. Interestingly, the foods we eat and how we supplement can have a significant impact on the brain. Each individual must be carefully considered and treated in an individualized manner. There is no one rule of thumb as to what supplements to take, and taking them haphazardly can have an adverse effect on many physiological processes. Consult with your medical professional before supplementing.

There are a few exceptions and recommendations for boosting brain power that everyone should consider, most of which is supported by Dr. David Perlemutter in his book Grain Brain:

1. For optimal health, we must take a quality probiotic daily to heal the gut and increase immunity. Illness, lack of sleep, and fatigue can increase the symptoms of stuttering.
2. Because we aren't getting enough omega 3's in the diet, and to decrease inflammation in the body, a high quality EPA/ DHA fish oil is recommended.
3. Vitamin C is important for everything from repairing and regenerating cells to preventing cancer.
4. B vitamins-energy vitamins (B6 especially), are essential for the synthesis of important chemicals, like serotonin, dopamine and norepinephrine. They are the energy vitamins.
5. Alpha Lipoic Acid- is a powerful antioxidant for the brain.
6. Turmeric-Another powerful antioxidant for the brain, also fights inflammation.
7. Last but not least, we are a society deficient in Vitamin D3. It's a necessary hormone and important for optimal health.

From the RDA example above, also consider a quality multi-vitamin without iron, even in a child's daily regimen. Vitamins without iron should be considered because iron can cause oxidative stress and inflammation in the brain, even suggesting it can contribute to mitochondrial decay. http://www.lef.org/Magazine/2012/3/Excess-Iron-Brain-Degeneration/Page-01

With nourishing foods and dietary supplements, we can begin a program of brain wellness.

Five

HEALING STUTTERING WITH QUALITY SPEECH
THERAPY AND NATURAL PHILOSOPHIES

What techniques do you believe will be beneficial in the treatment of stuttering?

1. What we say is as important as how we say it,
so say it in a thought provoking way.

I cannot imagine how difficult it would be to remember and implement a multitude of strategies before I was able to convey my thoughts. Many of my adolescent clients over the years get so frustrated that they just prefer to not talk at all at times. This can be very straining on relationships, and particularly on the self-esteem of the individual. I would like to see some simple strategies that can be more automatic and not require the continued focus on a list of strategies to basically "stutter in a more fluent way."

Let's begin with a rather simple strategy that I teach right from preschool ages; it is a strategy that creates more thoughtful individuals. It is so simple, you may even wonder why I am including this strategy, how-ever, research has shown that this simple strategy can create a more fluent student population. So get in the classrooms early and model critical thinking.

This simple strategy begins with a simple phrase, "Hmm, let me think about that," while looking up and placing a finger or a finger and thumb on your chin. As you get comfortable with the strategy, you can begin to fade parts of the strategy. Therefore, I may say "Hmm," and drop the rest of the statement, while still looking up and holding a finger on my chin. Next I will drop the finger on the chin, so I am still saying "Hmm" and looking up. For most students, you can even drop the "Hmm" and just look up, however for my dysfluent students; I keep the "Hmm" as a vocal warm up and to replace "um." Eventually, you may be even able to fade the "Hmm" and just think pause.

"Hmm" is a very important tell-ale sound. Where we say our "Hmm" reveals the pitch range most optimal for your voice. That's a good place to start. Often I find that my clients are not speaking at their optimal pitch. I hear the "um" "um" "um" from my clients who stutter, and then the voice follows at a pitch unrepresentative of the pitch of the "um." I may have my clients say "um-Hmm" to feel the difference in where the sound is located and solidify the optimal pitch. Saying "um" has no real air flow posture, and gets frequently repeated. "Hmm," on the other hand, is softer and lengthens the airflow emissions. It has a means of relaxing the vocal folds before speaking, where "um" can add a level of tension. "Um" requires movement of the oral postures, where "Hmm" does not. In ad-dition, when saying "um," it gives the appearance of being blocked or not sure of what you want to say. When you say "Hmm," it is a common and important way to make the statement that what you say is well thought out.

Think "Hmm…" Think pause.

2. What we say is as important as how we say it,
so lets be heard.

When visiting my clients in their homes, I was amazed by the occasions when they were fluent versus dysfluent, and I began to notice a pattern. When they were loud, as in cheering when their football team made a touchdown, they were fluent. When they sat at the dinner table and questions were flowing with their families, they were quiet and more dysfluent. Could they have a similar sensory issue that Parkinson's patients present with? Do individuals who stutter similarly think they are loud, when in fact they are actually soft spoken? Does being loud require increased respiratory support? Does being loud reduce laryngeal tension? This was an interesting observation, and one, which needed further exploration. The other factor we must consider here is that the cheers were automatic comments, whereas the questions proposed at the dinner table required volitional thought. Therefore, the more automatic one can be, the louder one can be, and the more breath to support utterances, the more opportunities we may have to be fluent. And the more fluent we are with these automatic comments, the greater chance fluency will carry over to all speech. In any event, it will certainly increase the confidence of the speaker.

This struck a personal note with me. When my mother was diagnosed with Parkinson's disease, I began focusing all my efforts on ways to help treat this disease and to help her maintain her voice. I found an interesting therapeutic approach that targeted increased vocal amplitude, sensory calibration, and had long-term maintenance voice treatment outcomes. The program was called the Lee Silverman Voice Treatment (LSVT), or LSVT LOUD. It was a therapeutic approach particularly for Parkinson's patients, and more recently has showed positive outcomes for patients with other neurological disorders. I am now a certified LSVT LOUD clinician.

"Focused on a single goal "speak LOUD!" – the treatment improves respiratory, laryngeal and articulatory function to maximize speech intelligibility."
http://www.lsvtglobal.com/patient-resources/what-is-lsvt-loud

Interestingly, in the conference I also learned that too little dopamine was associated with Parkinson's disease, and even more interestingly, that over 90% of individuals with Parkinson's had no genetic predisposition. This disorder was primarily the result of chemicals in the environment (or maybe even in our food supply) or was induced from medically prescribed or injected drugs. In my mom's case, she went in for surgery and woke up with Parkinson's disease.

The genes may have loaded the gun, but the pharmaceuticals pulled the trigger.

In addition to dopamine, norepinephrine is deficient in Parkinson's patients. "Norepinephrine is the chemical messenger to the sympathetic nervous system…which controls many automatic functions of the body."
http://nihseniorhealth.gov/parkinsonsdisease/whatcausesparkinsonsdisease/01.html

Can something similar possibly occur in stuttering? Within the area of stuttering are new medical findings, indicating that there is a common link, excess or interrupted dopamine, which is the exact opposite of Parkinson's. It would also seem likely that since dopamine is so closely related to norepinephrine, that excess or absent norepinephrine may exist. We also know that there can be a genetic predisposition to stuttering, as it has commonly run in families. If the older family members had stuttering that was minimal and resolved easily, but the child today faces more dramatic effects, what may be the cause? Hmm…can environmental toxins or medically prescribed or injected drugs have pulled the trigger?

Now let's look into environmental considerations and pharmaceuticals. There has been no stuttering research that I am aware of that considers the possibility of environmental toxins, including those in our food supply, and/or pharmaceutical toxins that we have ingested or have been injected into us. Being that children present with symptoms and are diagnosed at such a young age, the pharmaceutical toxins that they are exposed to are traditionally vaccines, which often contain mercury, formaldehyde, and even anti-freeze, and the list goes on. Dr. Boyd Haley stated that "A single vaccine given to a 6 pound infant is the equivalent of giving a 180 lb adult 30 vaccines." The link I have attached reveals not only the ingredient list in the vaccines given to our children, but the related side effects.

//healthwyze.org/index.php/component/content/article/60-vaccine-secrets. html Can environmental and pharmaceutical toxins play a role in the development or severity of stuttering? That is a question to be asked. Now let's look at the food supply and the environment. Cleaning supplies, flame retardants, plastics, fluoride in the water supply, GMO's, pesticides, insecticides...where does this end? In addition to the environmental and pharmaceutical toxins, we also have "sugar." We previously said that the average man, woman, and child in America eat about 150 pounds of sugar a year. Sugar causes dopamine levels to surge. Can sugar be a link? This is another question to be asked.

In *Grain Brain*, Dr. David Perlemutter states that,

"Sugar is a powerful brain toxin."

In addition to the similar medical factors, similar voice characteristics of Parkinson's patients may be present in some individuals who stutter. Although individuals who stutter have a preserved voice, do they also lack the sensory awareness of the stuttering? Do they lack the sensory awareness of amplitude? Do they use adequate breath support for speech? Both appear to speak softly.

Are individuals who stutter more aware of the reactions of others to their speech? These are all questions to be considered in the evaluation and treatment of this disorder.

Now consider the use of similar strategies, as in finding the optimal pitch, increasing the amplitude of what we say, increasing and using proper breath support, and increasing the sensory calibration of what we are saying, can we achieve more fluent speech? I am using these strategies currently and having some positive results. However, I would not even consider this approach in isolation, without correspondingly increasing optimal nutrition and targeting supplements to improve neurotransmitter function. In fact, remember that we started with improving overall physical health. The plan was optimal nutrition, neurotransmitter testing, and supplementation, followed by quality speech therapy. One of the quality speech therapy approaches that I recommend includes techniques (respiratory, laryngeal, and articulatory function) to increase vocal intensity, or even possibly a similar approach to LSVT "LOUD" techniques.

Think Loud!

3. What we say is as important as how we say it,
so put your best voice forth.

In addition to pitch and loudness, in the case of stuttering blocks, we often observe laryngeal tension. In the presence of blocks, airflow is too decreased to even permit phonation. Most intervention approaches to this issue are stuttering modification techniques- or behavioral approaches. These techniques focus on "management" of the disorder rather than "elimination" of the disorder. My focus here today takes a more naturalistic approach to eliminate the blocks in stuttering. There, I said it! If we treat the underlying cause, rather than the symptoms, our chance for a cure is possible.

There is observed laryngeal tension associated with blocks. I was in the theatre for many years, and particularly musical theatre. My art was mostly in my voice. Therefore, the same techniques an actor would use to achieve and maintain an optimal voice, are the same vocal health regimens I would determine to be appropriate for individuals who stutter. In theatre, I focused my vocal training on removing the tension in my vocal folds, focusing on orofacial resonance, and using adequate breath support. I warmed up the articulators and prepared myself to be heard. In theatre, everything I said and how I said it was important. In addition, we learn to reduce physical tension and techniques that support our optimal voice, and we practice vocal rest, get quality sleep, maintain adequate nutrition and hydration, perform regular vocal exercises, and practice calmness under pressure. The voice is just like any other muscle. Rather than managing stuttering or modifying behavior, lets take a positive approach. Let's put our best voice forth.

Think voice!

What alternative interventions or non-traditional healing tools
may be beneficial to treat stuttering?

How can Acupuncture possibly heal stuttering?

In Chinese medicine, acupuncture has been used for a host of disorders for thousands of years. Recently there has been increasing research showing that acupuncture may be a possible treatment in the case of stuttering. There are several acupuncture points relative to the causal and the symptomatic factors of this disorder. There is very limited research at this time; however I would be remiss to exclude this from the list of potential alternative interventions.

Consider Acupuncture!

What is EFT Tapping, and how can it help in improving stuttering?

A few years ago, I participated in the 2013 Tapping World Summit. The summit presented the philosophy of Emotional Freedom Techniques (EFT). The techniques are a form of tapping on the meridian acupressure points of Chinese acupressure, while employing the philosophies of modern psychology. The idea is to use your own body's energy and its magnificent power to heal while tapping on the meridian acupressure points. When we are in stressful situations, as faced by individuals who stutter, the flight or fight response in the body is activated. Cortisol eventually flat lines, and we see decreased neurotransmitters in the brain, particularly epinephrine and norepinephrine. There is a growing body of evidence today that supports the results of tapping in improving and even healing conditions that traditional medicine has failed to do.

In EFT, there are nine acupressure points that are stimulated, while at the same time, you face and accept yourself for who you are, problems and all. In this process, you reveal your true feelings about your problems, while sending calming signals to the brain, and letting the brain know you are safe and its okay to relax. How to tap and other information regarding this technique are best found at www.thetappingsolution.com. As a tapper myself, I would recommend taking the time to explore this technique. This is one area that will give the person who stutters and their families, a way to achieve acceptance, release the stress associated with stuttering, calm and relax the brain, and heal from anything that you are challenged by.

Consider EFT!

What is Earthing and how may it be beneficial to stuttering?

The Earth's energy is crucial for health. When we make direct contact with the Earth, we allow the Earth's energy to make us feel better. We now wear shoes and we live in buildings covered in concrete, wood, and carpet, with layers preventing us from connecting to the Earth. Since I moved from my home town Chicago to southern California, I spend lots of time walking barefoot on the beach. You become one with the Earth and the Earth's energy strengthens you. You feel better, look better, and even sleep better. Today because of the cooped up buildings and shoes and socks on our feet, we have to seek other ways to connect with the Earth's energy. This is called Earthing. It connects with the grounding port in your home, or the third hole in the outlet. Have you ever bought a grounding power strip, so that you could protect your television or computer for example? This same philosophy allows us to be grounded with the Earth. I bought my husband an Earthing mat for Christmas a few years back and he started sleeping on it every night. He noticed he was sleeping better, but he didn't realize how much. One night he went to sleep in the other room because he was getting sick and didn't want to get me sick. For several days he slept in the other room. He said his sleep was so interrupted, he never got a good night sleep and he felt awful. He blamed the lack of sleep on being sick, or just being in a different bed. All of a sudden he realized that he forgot his Earthing mat. Even being sick, the Earthing mat helped him get a good night's sleep. He told me that day he would never mistrust anything I told him. He is never without it. If something so simple can make you feel better, look better, and sleep better, it's all for me. The energy from the Earth makes me centered and in control. I find my creative forces rejuvenated. And, who doesn't like to look and feel better? Most important of all, I sleep better. These overall effects, particularly sleep, are extremely important to the person who stutters. Disrupted sleep creates a foggy brain, and we need the brain optimal to think and speak. We also need to emit a positive energy into the world around us.

"Allow the Earth's energy to strengthen you and help you sleep."

Consider Earthing!

Six

HEALING STUTTERING WITH PRIMARY FOODS

What does the inside look like? Here is an inside perspective:

Comments from a parent of one of my clients:

"My son has stuttered since first grade, and now he is a junior in high school. Stuttering is so challenging to deal with. He has attended speech therapy many different times in his life; he never wanted to go - it was very difficult and almost painful for him to go. He would immediately go from being happy to looking depressed that he had to go and deal with this issue. As he got older, it was more challenging, as he felt horrible that he had to go when most of the patients in the waiting room were kids much younger than him. I knew it was the right thing for him to do, but I hated to see him look so unhappy because of something I was making him do.

It is so hard to watch your child have a difficult time speaking the words that he wants to say. As a parent, I would worry about classmates making fun of him, his ability to have fun making and talking to friends, his ability to give school presentations, and ultimately his ability to interview for a job. I would do anything to help him with this problem."

To my parents of children who stutter:
I recognize that you have the utmost care and compassion for your child. I can truly say that you go over and above to follow any and all recommendations, even if they are out of the box to help improve your child. My hope is that my efforts will ease the worries and fears you face for your child, allow you to really know your child,
and celebrate the transformation you see as the healing begins.

Warmest thanks for all you do for your child.

From my client, her son:

"I have been stuttering for as long as I can remember. I have more trouble saying something first, rather than responding to someone. This makes me not want to start a conversation with someone, so I lose some friends that way. For example, I usually make friends in a semester and when the next semester comes, I don't want to have a conversation with them. Also, I don't want to try to make friends, since that would mean that I would have to start the conversation. Furthermore, my mom has made me go to a speech therapist for a long time. My speech improves with them, but once I stop seeing them, I start to stutter again. My tip with other people who have speech problems is for them to be gluten-free, speak louder and pause before talking. My speech got better once I started to try those things, but I'm still trying to pause more."

And to my clients:
May you believe in who you are. You are an individual first and foremost, who just happens to stutter. Trust in yourself and have the confidence to be the person you are. If you judge yourself, others will judge you. Show the world that judgment is unacceptable in any terms. If they choose not to be your friend, be sorry for them because they will miss out on knowing what an amazing individual you are.

Warmest thanks to you for the effort you put into healing yourself and for your trust in me to help you heal.

1. What about Primary Foods?

Relationships

Remember in Chapter 4 we spoke about the importance of primary foods as outlined by the Institute of Integrative Nutrition. They are the energy force within us and the force that makes us who we are. They are the positive and thriving relationships that we share, passionate student life and careers, strength and energy from physical exercise, and peace from the conventions of spirituality. Above you read the words of parent and child speaking from the heart, yet with some reservation for sharing this information to the world. The kind of compassion, challenges, and fears that parents experience when they see their child struggling in ways that the world treats so judgmentally, can tax even the most cherished relationships. Families can be divided, and even siblings struggle to understand. You heard the voice of the individual who stutters, and the overall challenges with being who they are and connecting with friends, family, and the world. This has a significant impact on overall health, because of the breakdown in these primary foods. As this individual is using some of the strategies I propose, such as going gluten free, pausing/thinking before speaking, and being louder, you hear a confidence in those words, as this individual makes this recommendation to others. This gives me great hope, as this individual must be finding some strength within himself to suggest or even recommend that what he is doing may work for others who stutter. It is my hope that confidence improves even more, so that the fear of connecting with friends and building friendships that strongly help us understand the world and how we fit into it, may find its way to a place of "courage." This is not to say that the person who stutters is not courageous. I know that every day it takes a tremendous amount of courage for the person who stutters, yet what I am saying is to center that courage and strength. Don't waste the courage on whether you will stutter when you get up, go to school, or in after school sports every day. Be courageous in those first words you utter to speak with someone. It was clear my client wanted to start new conversations and make new friends. If you want to do it, do just that. Don't stop life until the stuttering is "cured." We all are in a place of healing, yet we just don't wear our disorder so openly.

Also, did you know that only 25% of communication is verbal? Body language, facial expressions, and gestures make up 75% of all communication. Don't ever compromise who you are and what you want to do because saying the first word is hard. You can make the first word non-verbal. Smile, wave, make eye contact, and lean in closely. These non-verbal moves all say way more than the word, "hello." Now, you have removed the challenge of the first word. You don't always need to connect with a word.

What you need to do is: "CONNECT."

Another thought.....
There is someone out there, who is just waiting to know "YOU." My dad always said that if you have one true friend in your life, you are a lucky person. Every time you meet someone new, think to yourself, "this may be my best friend," and give it a chance. Don't ever be afraid to make the first move or speak the first word, even when it gets stuck, because every time you do, you are feeding those

primary foods, you are achieving improved health, and you are achieving the cure you seek so desperately. You may even be making a best friend!

Student Life/ Career

Whether you are out in the work force, or a youthful student, find something you are passionate about. Living a life filled with passion is living life. If you are afraid to speak, afraid to make the first move, afraid to be who you are, the chance of finding that passion will be challenging. When you are thinking about what you want to do, or a project in an exciting class, I beg of you, put that first. Your excitement in what you are doing will be far greater an energy force than anything else you can do to improve fluency.

Find the passion in what you do.

Exercise

Exercise, provides strength not only for the body, but for the neurotransmitters in the brain. Are you aware that exercise stimulates serotonin? They always say that individuals who exercise are happy people. There are lots of forms of exercise. If you are in school, take on a sport. There is a social benefit as well as an exercise benefit. Consider yoga, an exercise that strengthens the body and relaxes the brain. Exercise builds energy for the challenges we face in life, and don't we all need more of that in this hectic world?

Build energy and strengthen mood with exercise.

There are other forms of exercise. For example, actors exercise before they speak. They "get ready to speak." The individual who stutters is not unlike the actor.

I recommend you do it like the professionals do. Exercise helps with breath support for speech. It helps reduce overall tension in the body, and exercising the articulators (parts of the mouth that form speech sounds) helps you reduce tension in speech and gets you ready to speak. You can stretch away tension and warm up the motor system for movement. As you exercise, the strength in your body supports vocal resonance, and the combination of breath and resonance supports loudness and maintaining the quality of the loudness.

For improved fluency, exercise the body and the articulators.

Exercise for energy, for strength, and for speech.

Spirituality

Whether you believe in God, or you see something bigger and better in nature, or you meditate, or you even find grace within yourself, we all need to find a sense of goodness, grace, and serenity in the world we live in. Life can be challenging for us all, and taking that time, centers you. When the world seems overwhelming, particularly for the person who stutters, take some time to remove yourself from the situation and gain perspective.

Find yourself, find goodness, find peace.

Health Coaching

What is a Health Coach?

A Health Coach is an inspirational wellness authority who provides motivation and support in helping others achieve optimal wellness and health through nutrition and lifestyle choices. Health Coaches provide increasing awareness for what health really is and are essential to help others achieve optimal health and well-being. As a Health Coach myself, I am blessed to be part of a profession where I can use all my talents and energy in making a positive difference in the world.

What are the benefits of working with a Health Coach to improve stuttering?

With the new findings in stuttering related to the neurotransmitters in the brain, and the side effects of the pharmaceutical management of this disorder, it makes sense that we consider a more natural approach such as "food as medicine." Health Coaches can assist individuals who stutter with nutritional guidance, as well as support balancing lifestyle aspects of optimal health. In my personal opinion, even more than the nutritional aspects of nourishing the brain, it is the lifestyle aspects that are severely deficient in most individuals who are dysfluent. It has been heart breaking to hear the accounts of individuals who stutter and the sense of isolation they must feel.

*With the support of a Health Coach,
you will learn that the power to heal is within you.*

Remember that food is medicine, lifestyle considerations are within your reach, and hopefully this book will give you the wisdom to achieve radiant wellness in your life. What a sense of empowerment that will be for you!

Consider a Health Coach for optimal health and overall well-being.

Things to consider…

As you reflect on the sense of wellness you will achieve with mindfulness and balance in your life, there are a few simple things to remember and an exercise that will help you define exactly what is important to you. As you reflect on the following and begin the exercise, take time to really look at yourself and affirm that you have the power within yourself to heal. Only then will you find the freedom to be who you are.

Remember that...

...It only takes a few seconds to breathe just a few breaths.

...It only takes a few seconds to stop the negative feeling in your brain. Visualize what you don't want to see with a big red line through it. Then visualize what you do want to see and spray it pink.

...It only takes a few seconds to make an affirmation. Remember EFT. Affirm that you can handle any situation, even stuttering.

...It only takes a few seconds to ground yourself. Stand tall and be one with the Earth.

...it only takes a few seconds to realize you are not alone. Don't be afraid to consider a Health Coach to guide you in your journey of healing along with a speech pathologist.

...it only takes a few seconds to "love yourself up!"

And in each of those few seconds, you will begin to realize the importance of balance in your life. You will have the clarity and peace of mind to not allow stuttering to be the driving force of your life. You won't make each day about whether you stuttered or didn't stutter because you will have found what's important in your life. You will seek what's important. You will have found how to balance your life and to accept who you are with all your imperfections.

At the Institute of Integrative Nutrition, they use something called the Circle of Life to increase awareness of balance in your primary foods. It has 12 sections-joy, spirituality, creativity, finances, career, education, health, physical activity, home cooking, home environment, relationships, and social life. They use an exercise where you plot points on the circle near the center for areas in your life that you are dissatisfied with and on the periphery for things you have achieved ultimate happiness in. When you connect the dots, you will have your personal Circle of Life. You will be able to identify imbalances in your life so that you can be more focused on areas you want to improve. For some individuals who stutter, the Stuttering Circle of Life seems to be 2 sections, comprised of "stuttering" and "not stuttering."

I have included the link for the Circle of Life Exercise presented by Integrative Nutrition.

http://www.integrativenutrition.com/circleoflife

Create your personal Circle of Life. Fill each section with things that are personally important to you and plot your points. Only then, will you see what you need to balance for happiness and joy in your life.

Find your balance in life!

Wrapping up primary foods:

Feed yourself. Feed the primary foods in a nourishing way just as you do the secondary foods. Be who you are and never let anyone or anything take that away from you. And don't be afraid to seek guidance along the way.

You are an Individual first, who just happens to stutter. Don't make stuttering who you are. It doesn't deserve the top billing over you.

Seven

BRINGING IT ALL TOGETHER
SEVEN STEPS TO BEING A FLUENT
SPEAKER FOR LIFE!

Before beginning this program, it is my recommendation that any child or individual who experiences dysfluency to any degree be assessed by a qualified speech and language pathologist to rule out any co-existing or in-fluencing speech and language disorder. With this knowledge, the influence of other factors may be remediated and the fluency may improve. We see this from the comments of the group of speech pathologists that were consider-ate enough to contribute to this process. To the individuals who experience dysfluency that persists even with treatment, consider seeking the support of a speech and language pathologist who supports your personal philosophy. We saw that treatment is often behavioral or even can be pharmaceutical. If one approach isn't working for you, seek the philosophy or the approach that will. In addition, because of the influence of environmental chemical hazards and a food and water supply that is pesticide and insecticide loaded, I encourage you to seek the support of a health coach. Consider taking a personal stand on the pharmaceuticals you ingest or what you will allow to be injected into you.

Trust that you are not controlled by your genes or defined by your disorder. You are not your disorder. Don't let the dysfluency be all that you are.

Be the best "YOU" that you can be, fluent or not, and don't ever feel like you have to do it alone.

Release the bonds of stuttering by rewiring how you think!

1.   Rewire the brain with real food.
Consider rediscovering real foods- vegetables, fruits, meats, eggs, real dairy, and whole (gluten free) grains. *Forget the whites and fill your life with color!*

2.   Rewire the brain with knowledge.
We have the ability to see exactly what's going on in the brain. Insist on neurotransmitter testing, so that when you are healing you aren't shooting in the dark.

3.   Rewire the brain with quality supplements.
Once you know the areas of weakness in the brain, work with a qualified health coach or natural medical provider to combine foods and supplements to achieve an optimal brain. Just as with hormones, we don't want to be in the typical "range," we want to be optimal at all times.

4.   Rewire the brain with quality speech therapy.
Rule out co-existing or influencing disorders.
New ideas-Think Hmmm…, think LOUD, think breath, and think voice.

5.   Rewire the brain with alternative therapies.
Consider acupuncture, EFT, and Earthing. Consider anything, no matter if the world thinks you are crazy, which will make you a confident and happier individual.

6. Rewire the brain with primary foods.
Remember that you are a person, an amazing person, who just happens to stutter. You are not a "stutterer," and don't ever respond to that label. You are so many other things. Celebrate your relationships and seek new ones. Center yourself and establish your optimal mood with exercise. Challenge yourself in school or in work and be passionate in all you do. Last but not least, find the grace and beauty in the world and within yourself.

7. Rewire the brain by putting yourself first.
Right now, it's all about you. "Love yourself up," is a phrase I heard often in my health coaching education by Joshua Rosenthal, at the Institute of Integrative Nutrition, and I use it frequently in my practice. Let me say it again, "Love Yourself Up." You need to love yourself, believe in yourself, and have confidence in yourself, before the world will love you, too. This is important for us all to remember.

Here's to freedom from stuttering!

Celebrate who you are.
Celebrate a life well lived.
Celebrate the differences between us…
until difference no longer makes a difference…

Patricia

Resources

Books to Read:

1. Grain Brain, by Dr. David Perlmutter
2. *In Defense of Food,* by Michael Pollan
3. *Simply Sugar Free,* by Sue Brown
4. *10-Day Detox*, Dr. Mark Hyman
5. *J. J. Virgin's Sugar Impact Diet,* by J. J. Virgin
6. *Deep Nutrition, Why Your Genes Need Traditional Food*, by Catherine Shannahan
7. *What Color is Your Diet,* by David Heber MD
8. *The Adrenal Reset Diet,* Dr. Alan Christianson

Where to Find Books on Stuttering
The Stuttering Foundation. Web. http://www.stutteringhelp.org/books-stuttering

Neurotransmitter Testing
Pharmasan Labs. Web. http://www.pharmasan.com/

Work Cited

Chapter 1
Stuttering Facts and Information. The Stuttering Foundation, 1991-2015. Web. http://www.stutteringhelp.org/faq

Medical Aspects of Stuttering. Riley, Glyndon. California State University, 2002. Web. http://www.stutteringhelp.org/medical-aspects-stuttering

Stuttering. ASHA, 1997-2015. Web. http://www.asha.org/public/speech/disorders/stuttering.htm#a

Chapter 2
What Speech-Language Pathologists Need to Know About the Emerging Medical Treatments in Stuttering (Ep. 429). Maguire, Dr. Gerald, Nov. 2013. Web http://stuttertalk.com/tag/gerald-maguire/

Treating the School-Age Child Who Stutters. Ramig, Peter R. University of Colorado. Web. http://www.stutteringrecovery.com/childinterv.PDF

Chapter 3:
Perlmutter, Dr. David Grain Brain, Little, Brown and Company, 2013 Print.

Are GMO's Safe. Kresser, Chris. Web. http://chriskresser.com/are-gmos-safe

Chapter 4
Color Me Healthy-Eating for a Rainbow of Benefits, Schaeffer, Juliann Today's Dietician Vol. 10 No. 11 P. 34 2015. Web. http://www.todays-dietitian.com/newarchives/110308p34.shtml://www.todaysdietitian.com/newarchives/110308p34.shtml

What Are Neurotransmitters? Neurogistics 2014. Web. https://www.neurogistics.com/TheScience/WhatareNeurotransmi09CE.asp

Chapter 5
Ortner, Nick The Tapping Solution. Hay House Publishing, 2013 Print

Reducing Laryngeal Tension During Stuttering. Coleman Craig 2015. http://www.speechpathology.com/ask-the-experts/reducing-laryngeal-tension-during-stuttering-1087

What is LSVT Loud LSVT Global. Web. http://www.lsvtglobal.com/patient-resources/what-is-lsvt-loud

Chapter 6
Primary Food
http://www.integrativenutrition.com/blog/2008/03/26/primary-food
Integrative Nutrition

The Circle of Life Exercise
http://www.integrativenutrition.com/circleoflife

www.ingramcontent.com/pod-product-compliance
Lightning Source LLC
Chambersburg PA
CBHW070911280326
41934CB00008B/1677